MICHELLE ROBINSON

Guide For Touring A Nursing Home

TIPS ON PICKING THE BETTER FACILITY

First edition

This book was professionally typeset on Reedsy.
Find out more at reedsy.com

Contents

1

INTRODUCTION

My name is Michelle Robinson and my goal is to attempt to give you an idea of what to look for while taking a tour of a nursing home. Nursing homes have many different terms such as long term care, SNF (skilled nursing facility, pronounced as sniff), convalescent home, or for a lack of better names "old folks home".I strongly dislike the term "old folks home"! The term is used by the older generations. The purpose of the book is not to make you an expert on taking a tour, but to assist in bringing awareness to identifying safety and good quality care for your loved one.

Just a little about myself. I have been caring for the elderly since I was 15 years old. It started with taking care of my great grandmother (Ala Bama) when she became ill with double pneumonia. Yes, her real name is Ala Bama. My grandmother (Clara Faye) was working a full time job and was taking care of my grandfather who had lung cancer. When my great grandmother became ill with double pneumonia ,my grandmother was going to have to place her in a nursing home. The care of two dependent ill people and a full time job was more than she could handle alone. My mom and dad decided to bring my great grandmother to our home and care for her.This is how I started taking care of the elderly at 15 years old.

One night, after I helped my great grandmother to the bedside commode, she had a massive heart attack right in front of my eyes. Being 15 years old I did the only thing I knew to do. I ran to my parents room screaming "HELP,HELP, something is wrong with Granny". My parents and I went to her room and my dad called 911 to activate the emergency response team. Unfortunately my granny did not make it. She was flown by helicopter to the hospital. Once she was in the helicopter they were able to revive her. When the helicopter was en route to the hospital, she had her 2nd massive heart attack and passed away. Because I did not know how to help my Granny, I realized that my purpose was to become a nurse and help the elderly.

I have been a nurse for 22 years. I was a CNA (certified nursing assistant) for 6 years prior to becoming a nurse..I have gained experience and knowledge in the long term care industry. I have taught C.N.A.classes. I have been a wound care nurse. I have even been an A.D.O.N.(Assistant Director of Nurses). The only thing I have not done (within my scope of practice) is be a M.D.S. nurse(the nurse that bills for the work that the facility does). I have such a passion for the elderly that it gets me in trouble sometimes. What I mean by that is I am the biggest resident advocate you will ever meet. I love the elderly with all my heart and my soul. I believe they should be given dignity and respect ALWAYS! Just because they require assistance with ADLs (activities of daily living) does not mean they have to do what everyone tells them.This also includes you. They are still adults. They have rights in long term care.I will list their rights towards the end of this book. Understand, these rights are mandated by the Centers for Medicare and Medicaid Services. This is a government office. "Resident" is a term that is used in long term care meaning basically the person that lives in the facility.

My goal is to attempt to give you some understanding on things to look for on a tour of a facility. Knowledge is power! This book is just the beginning on how I feel that I can serve the elderly. I feel by educating the families and nursing home staff that I can reach more of the elderly population, raise awareness and put back to compassion then what I can in person.

In 2019, my grandmother (Clara Faye age 85) made the decision to place herself in a long term care facility. I asked her to live where I worked. Over my years of geriatric nursing I felt at peace with her decision because I was trained and ready for what was to come. She passed away in 2020 on hospice services with dignity and respect.

LET'S GET INTO IT!

2

PREPARING FOR THE TOUR

Finding a facility can sometimes be FRUSTRATING and STRESSFUL. First you should determine what type of facility you will need. There is some safety awareness that I need to point out. I am going to attempt to do this as gently as I can. I am by no means trying to be negative towards nursing homes. There are a lot of GREAT homes out there. There are also bad nursing homes out there. Every elderly person's situation is different. If your loved one has been diagnosed with Dementia, Alzheimer and is a wanderer then there is a specific type of facility you might need. If your loved one is alert and oriented to place, time, situation then their needs will be different. It is all about safety.There are facilities that have what is called a "locked unit" or a "memory care unit". The purpose of a locked unit is to keep them safe. It is not a behavior unit. A Lot of people don't have this understanding. The purpose of a locked unit is because the resident wanders outside with no safety awareness. For example: an elderly person may be very demented and does not have the cognitive ability to know that if they step in front of a moving car they will get hit. It's about safety not behavior. I

4

also want to bring awareness that a locked unit is only locked to a certain point. There are life safety codes mandated by the state that the facility has to maintain. For example if the resident pushes and holds the door that is "locked" for 15 seconds, the door will release.This has to be in place in case there is a fire so your loved one may exit the unit to get to safety.These types of units have a keypad with a numerical code to enter the unit. But know that an alarm will sound very loudly to alert staff that the resident is attempting to open the door. They should respond very quickly. Some facilities have what is called a "wander guard system". This is not a secured unit, but serves somewhat the same purpose. This system also has a very loud alarm to alert staff that a resident is attempting to get outside of the facility. In order for this system to function properly the resident has to have what is called a "wander guard bracelet". Depending on the type of system, if they get close to the sensor it alarms but most commonly used is where the resident has to actually push on the door for the alarm to sound. So with that said, it is important to know the location of the facility. If you are unsure about the type of facility it's okay. When you go for a tour make sure you ask the person touring you. This question would be a good question for the Director of Nursing. This is what you can say "I am not sure if my loved one needs a secure unit or not. Can you help me determine if they need a secure unit?" They should ask you some simple easy questions about your loved one's behaviors in the home setting.

Back to searching for facilities. I prefer to use the google search engine. As I mentioned earlier, there are many names that are used for nursing homes. I recommend starting your search with " long term care" or "skilled nursing facility". Write down the facilities that peak your interest. I would recommend at least 5-6 facilities. I recommend using one blank sheet of paper for each facility you have chosen. At the top of the page write the facility name, address and phone number. Write these words: Administrator, Director of Nurses and Person touring. Make sure you leave space to write their name. Also write this word: Ombudsman. I will explain later about this. As you are looking on the internet for facilities, I recommend reading some of the reviews. While reading reviews keep in mind, negative reviews are not always written by family members or even residents of that facility. Sometimes disgruntled employees write bad reviews based on their employment. Don't mark a facility off your list because of some bad reviews. Just make a mental note.

Now that you have 5-6 facilities you have picked out, it's time to set up your tour. I would recommend you tour during the times I am about to list.

If you have to tour during the morning time then choose any time after 10:30 am. The reason you do not want to go earlier then 10:30 am is because if you have questions for the Director of Nurses, they are typically in meetings until then. You want their undivided attention. It also shows respect. Those meetings are very important. The Department Managers start with what is called "Stand up". This is where the entire IDT (Interdisciplinary Team,)meets to discuss what is going on in the facility on a day to day basis. Ensuring that the resident's needs are being met. You will not want to try and tour a facility after 3:30 PM. This is because after 3:30 PM everyone is busy trying to wrap up their day so they can leave at 5:00 PM. They will be busy and you may/may not be rushed through your tour. These are just recommendations to get the most out of your tour.

Now, call the facilities and schedule a tour. When scheduling make sure you get the person's name that will be giving you a tour. Write the date and time for that facility. Life happens and you could forget. So write the date and time on the proper facility paper. Moving forward I will refer to the person giving the tour as your "tour guide". Make sure you allow for at least an hour for each tour. I say this because you will have questions and those answers might lead into other questions. So allowing at least an hour I feel that you will get the best experience possible. I am not saying the tours are going to be an hour long.Also, ask if the Director of Nurse and the Administrator will be in the building for the day you will be touring. Make sure you get their names and write it on the paper for that facility. Keep in mind life happens.They may have a family emergency or have gotten sick and are unable to be in the building on your tour. If that happens, it's okay, I have not run across any Director of Nurses or Administrator that wont answer your questions by phone. Just leave your name and number with your tour guide. **Make sure you are not late for your tour.** You will have a better experience if you are on time. They may have more than one tour scheduled for the day. I recommend **you arrive approximately 10-15 minutes** early. Sometimes if they don't have a tour scheduled then they will start your tour early. I do not recommend doing tours back to back. If you are in a bind and need to find a facility ASAP I would recommend doing no more than two tours a day. You will need a moment to process what you have heard and saw during your tour. If you are in a bind, I recommend touring one before lunch and one after lunch.Make sure you get directions to the facility. Be familiar with the route you will take. This will help you to adjust on the time to get to the facility safely and on time. For example heavy traffic. All depends on where you live.

Make sure you write any questions you want to ask on the facility paper that you are touring **before** you tour. After your first tour, for the next tour you can write the same questions but you will probably have more questions to add based on your first tour. You will think of things also as you go along the tour. Write down everything you can.

3

THINGS TO BRING ON TOUR

You will need a pen or pencil. You will need paper. I recommend having a regular size spiral notebook. This way you will have a hard surface to write on your paper as you tour. Benefits of a spiral notebook are you will not have loose papers and you will always have all facility notes with you. Make sure you have the correct paper for the facility you are touring. Also bring your attention to detail. Attention to detail is your most valuable possession.

4

WHAT TO EXPECT ON YOUR TOUR

Okay we have set the date and time. Now the day is here for the tour. Here are some things you will typically see on a tour of a nursing home.

1. You will probably enter the facility through the front entrance. You should see a receptionist. Check in with this person. Just tell them you have an appointment to tour the facility with whomever is doing your tour. The receptionist will most likely ask you to have a seat while they let the touring person know you are there. As you are sitting waiting, this is a great opportunity to start looking at things.
2. Is the area free from clutter?
3. Is the floor clean
4. Is the area chaotic
5. Are there pamphlets displayed about the facility? I would recommend looking at one while you wait. Once your tour guide comes, ask them if you may have the pamphlet.

Typically they are free.I recommend taking a pamphlet from each facility you tour so that it will help remind you of the facility. There is typically good information in those about the facility and services offered.

So now your tour guide is here. Every facility is different on what order they do their tour. But basically they all typically show the following things. They will show what's called a showroom, the therapy gym, dining room(s), activity room, and common areas. I am going to talk a little about each of them.

SHOW ROOM

This is a room that is strictly set up for tours. It's not that they are attempting to put on a show. There are laws such as HIPAA that protect the residents that are already living there. Please respect the residents that are currently living there. The showroom is just to give you an idea about how the room may look. Sometimes the rooms look different. Especially if a resident is coming in for what nursing homes call "skilled services". There are two types of residents in long term care. There are long term residents which are typically permanently placed in a facility. There are short term residents which are people that just need therapy or nursing skilled services. Short term residents"skilled services" typically get what they need from nursing or therapy and return home. So the long term care rooms may be different than the short term rooms. The showroom is just to give you an idea of how the room looks.

THERAPY GYM

Typically this area is set aside away from resident's rooms. There are multiple disciplines in therapy. Such as PT (Physical therapy), OT (Occupational therapy and ST (Speech therapy).

Therapists teach the residents how to perform their activities of daily living according to their ability. Whether it is maintaining balance, dressing, brushing teeth or learning how to talk again. This helps promote independence. Promoting independence is a big deal.Residents should be encouraged to be as independent as possible.

Therapy gym you will see equipment. One thing to look for is that the floor does not have items laying on the floor. Are there clear pathways for the resident to walk? Does the gym have an inviting appearance? If there are residents in the gym, do they look comfortable? Do they appear in distress? Are the therapists engaged with the residents? Sometimes residents perform exercises that do not require the therapist to be right beside them. Just look at the environment and think "would my loved one enjoy the therapy gym or does it look like it is a chore?" Therapy gyms are typically fun for the residents. Even though they are exercising and learning, Therapist are creative and have big personalities that make exercising and learning fun!

DINING ROOM(S)

When being shown the dining room(s) note if the area is clean.

Is there a TV in the dining room? Look around to see if they have coffee or other fluids available. Common examples of fluids would be tea or water. Look and see if the tables are clean. Are there a lot of dirty dishes sitting around? Is the floor clean? Are the empty chairs pushed under the tables or scattered throughout the dining room? This could potentially create a fall risk for residents that walk with/without walkers. Is the dining room close to the kitchen? If the dining rooms are in a different place than the kitchen, how do the residents get served? I have worked in different facilities where dining rooms are next to the kitchen. I have also worked where the dining room is not close to the kitchen. The trays were transported from the kitchen to the dining room via cart. This just kind of helps you get an idea of how they will be served.

ACTIVITY ROOM

Some facilities have a designated area for small(approximately 4-5 people)group activities. Typically activities are done in the dining room. But if they do show you an activity room, look to see if the floor is free of clutter? Is there room for residents to be in there and not be crowded. The activity director is required to post their monthly calendar of activities. You may ask to see the calendar of activities. This is not private information. I suggest you take a look at it and see what type of activities they offer. Yes, residents love bingo but this should not be the only activity they offer. Outside of holidays, a good activity director will have those special activities to celebrate within a specific month. For example, February contains Valentine's Day. It is also Black History month. November is not only for Thanksgiving but

Veterans Day is in that month.Just look around on the calendar and see what they are doing. The calendar should be posted either outside the activity department or on the wall where all residents can see it.

COMMON AREAS

Common areas are where residents can go and hang out. Some facilities use a common area for storing books. The resident can pick a book to sit and read. Some common areas may contain an artificial fireplace. Some facilities have an area for the resident to visit with family. Sometimes the residents have roommates and a family may want to have alone time with their loved one. The common areas should be free of clutter and not have things lying around that could cause a resident to fall.

NURSES STATION(S)

Every facility is different when it comes to nurses stations. I have worked at facilities that had one nurses station. I have worked at a facility that had 4 nurses stations. It all depends on the size and the layout of the facility.

These are just some basic things that you may see during your tour. I have personally given tours of facilities that I have worked. I have never been a tour guide in a full time position. I focused on areas that are standard things

5

MEET SOME OF THE STAFF

FRONT LINE STAFF

There are many departments to a nursing home but, at this moment I am focusing on departments that come in direct contact with the residents the majority of the time. This is by NO MEANS saying one department is better than the other. Ever heard the expression "it takes a village to raise a child?". Every department is VERY important to the success of a nursing home.NO one department is superior to the other. The departments with the most interaction with all residents are Dietary, Housekeeping, Laundry , Maintenance and Nursing. Note that every department has a Department manager. I am referring to the people that work under these managers.

DIETARY: preps resident's meals and snacks. Dietary handles any food issues that might arise. For example, food likes and dislikes. **Meal substitutions. Need to know if your loved one does not like what is served can they get an alternative preference.**

HOUSEKEEPING: keeps the resident's room and bathroom clean. They also replenish toilet paper and paper towels in the bathroom. Basically generalized housekeeping. These hard workers are not just limited to resident rooms. They clean the ENTIRE building on a daily basis! Thank you to all the Housekeepers!

LAUNDRY: If you do not wish to do your loved one's laundry, the facility will do it for you. **This service should be included and not an extra charge.**The laundry staff is not limited to just the resident's clothing. They take care of any washing and drying needs for the facility. For example: towels, wash cloths, linen, dietary rags and many other needs by the need of the facility. Thank you to the Laundry staff!

MAINTENANCE: Maintenance is exactly what it means. The maintenance department maintains any repairs and the little tasks that a resident might need. A task may include hanging the new TV you bought for them on the wall or maybe the head of their bed won't go up.They keep everything in working order.Thank you to the Maintenance staff! **Speaking of TVs, you may want to ask your tour guide if the facility furnishes televisions or is the resident responsible for furnishing their own. This is facility based.**

NURSING:Nursing has many disciplines within the department. There are three main disciplines. You have CNAs, CMAs and Nurses. Let me tell you about these disciplines.**CNA**(Certified Nursing Assistant) These people are the ones that will eventually know your loved one the most. CNAs are the backbone of the Nursing department hands down! They are the ones that are assisting your loved one with their activities of daily living. From assisting with toileting needs(or incontinent care), bathing, brushing teeth, brushing hair, dressing and even feeding the residents that can not feed themselves. The aids are the ones that work the hardest. As a nurse, if my CNA comes and tells me something is wrong with a resident, I rush to go assess the resident. Nine times out of ten they are not wrong. Even with the slight change in mental status,just the slightest increase in confusion,the aids will identify it before any other staff in the building.They are the ones that spend the most with your loved one. CNAs are the most unappreciated people in the industry. A standing ovation is given to all of the CNAs out there! I see you all!

CMA(Certified Medication Aides) These people are CNAs that took a course,become certified to pass medication. This discipline is also overlooked. I, as a nurse, love it when I have a medication aide to pass my medications. It allows me to focus more on the residents health needs.

NURSES(LVN/LPNs and RNs) As a nurse myself, I have told you the story of how and why I became a geriatric nurse. My job is to ensure that CNAs and CMAs are doing their job. As a nurse, we are to ensure that the resident is getting needs met. Nurses have their own duties that they are responsible for like blood sugar checks and wound care. There are so many more duties involving a nurse.

Now I have kind of set the stage for the tour. Lets keep going.

6

TIME TO PAY ATTENTION TO DETAILS

As you are being walked through out the facility with your guide, Try to keep in mind some of the following:

THE STAFF'S FACES

When you are doing your tour, look at the staff faces as you pass them on your tour. Do they look like they are happy to be there? Do they say "Hello" or "Hi" as you pass them during your tour? Try saying "hello" or "Hi" to them. Maybe they are just shy. One of the ways to tell if a person is happy or glad to be there is they will speak back. Keep in mind though,that sometimes a staff gets so task focused that they may not hear you. They do have a lot of things to do and only 8 hours to complete them. Don't be offended if they do not speak. Just make a note for the next facility tour. You may see a difference with each facility.

THE RESIDENTS

As you are taking your, tour you will see residents. A few things to take into consideration are:

Does the resident look happy?

Is the resident's hair brushed?

Is there food on the resident's clothing? Make sure you take into consideration the time. If it is after lunch you have to give staff time to make their rounds. They typically have approximately 10-15 resident's each. The resident to CNA ratio is different for every facility.

If you can see a resident's fingernails, note if they are clean? You cant walkover and just be like "let me see your fingernails". But from a distance you sometimes can see if they are long or short. You sometimes can see dirt under the nails.Are the wheelchair or walker dirty?

ODORS

Is there foul odors? Now I need to elaborate on this subject. Understand that it is NOT normal that nursing homes have a continuous foul odor. A misunderstood understanding is that it is common for a nursing home to smell like urine and feces. **This is so far from the truth!** There are times that there may be the smell of urine or feces. But, those odors should not linger. These odors typically occur when CNAs make their rounds to check and change the residents due to incontinence. Once they have completed their round and taken out the trash, the odors should go away. I am not saying that there will never be any odors. What I am saying is if you are touring a facility and you smell a foul odor like feces or urine,it is okay to ask your tour person if the staff is making rounds at that time. You should definitely not smell feces in the dining room if residents are eating! The dining room should smell like food! This should raise a flag for you. Either one or two things have happened. Either a resident has had an incontinent episode while eating or the resident was brought to the dining room incontinent. In either situation, staff should assist the resident to their room and provide incontinent care immediately. A resident should not sit in their own feces while attempting to eat. That is so wrong on so many levels!

HALLWAYS

As you are touring, look down the hallways. The hallways should not be cluttered with wheelchairs, walkers,oxygen con-centrators or Hoyer lifts. The hallways should have a clear path. The hallways should have handrails on both sides of the hall.Handrails being present is for resident safety. Handrails allow the residents to walk the hallway while maintaining balance. This helps reduce falls. Now during rounds by the CNAs there may be a linen cart and barrels on the hallway. Those items should not be stored there when they are not making rounds.Everything has a place to be stored. It is not in the hallway!

BATHROOM

When looking at the showroom make sure you look at the bathroom. Make sure the bathroom has grab bars. These bars assist with independence and safety. There should be grab bars by the toilet and in the shower.

7

THINGS YOU SHOULD ASK

1. **Know what is available.**
2. Pharmacy: Know what pharmacy the facility uses. It is convenient for the facility and best interests the resident and family to use the same I am now going to give you some ideas of things that you can ask your tour guide. These are things that you should know and I will give an explanation of why you should know. Keep in mind that every facility is different.
3. Visiting hours: First and foremost once a person becomes a resident at a facility, it becomes their home. You should be able to visit your loved one as you would if they were still at home. I would be kind of leary if a facility had designated visiting hours. Now, if your loved one is a night owl and you would visit them at night, please be respectful of other residents. In other words, try not to be loud at 8:00 pm. I would recommend taking your loved one to a common area to visit. Now if your loved one is in a private room,

then close the door so that you may have privacy and your visitation will not disturb other residents within the home.

4. Television: As I mentioned in the Maintenance section of this book, you will need to find out if the facility furnishes televisions in the rooms. Some facilities do and some don't but that is something you will have to ask your tour guide.

5. Cable: Ask your tour guide if the facility provides cable or if the resident has to provide it themselves. Most facilities I have worked at provide basic cable. I have worked at a facility where a resident preferred satellite over cable. The facility allowed the resident to have a satellite dish placed on a pole outside of their window. But there again, that was 100% at the expense of the resident and family.

6. Internet: Ask if the facility provides WiFi internet access to the resident. Most facilities do. Some residents like to play games on a tablet or read an e book on their electronic device.

7. Phone: Some facilities have a phone in the resident's room. This is also facility based. Most homes, if they do not provide a phone in the resident's room, have a way for the resident or family to provide a phone. For example, at the family's or resident's expense they may have a landline put in room. There are some facilities that provide a phone in a resident's room. Just ask, your tour guide will know. If they don't know, they can find out for you.

8. Refrigerator: Most facilities allow residents to have a mini refrigerator in their room. Typically this is supplied by the resident or family. Sometimes residents like to have special drinks and snacks kept in their room. Let's just admit it..... Vending machine inflation is through the roof.

9. Microwaves: Most facilities will not allow microwaves

in resident's rooms for many reasons. The two biggest reasons are 1. Another resident may have a pacemaker and too close to a microwave and short out the pacemaker. 2. Residents can receive burns or set a microwave on fire, due to cognitive deficits. The facility typically has microwaves that the staff can heat up thighs for the resident.

10. Showering: As most facilities, showers in the rooms depend on what type of care they are needing. What I mean is long term care residents typically do not have a shower in their room unless they are privately paid. Private pay means they are paying for a private room either through their insurance company or out of pocket. Now most facilities have what is called a skilled unit. The skilled unit typically has private rooms with private showers. These rooms are for the residents that are there to receive their therapy or skilled nursing and go back home. An example of skilled nursing would be if they were to get IV antibiotics or wound care. You just need to ask your tour guide so you have a clear understanding.

11. Religious/Cultural Support: Ask your tour guide what kind of religious and cultural support they offer. Tell your tour guide some background on your loved one, For example, your loved one may enjoy group bible study. You want to make sure that a facility can meet all needs of your loved one.

12. Meal options: Does the facility offer an alternative meal at mealtimes in the event they don't like what is served? This is an important question also. Not all facilities offer an alternate meal.

13. In-house services: Ask your tour guide what in-house services they have available. This would be along the line of

having a podiatrist come to the facility. These are specialty doctors that facilities utilize. Typically podiatrist and ophthalmologist come quarterly. This is approximately every 3 months. Some facilities offer psychiatric services. I worked in a facility where they had a Nurse Practitioner that worked under a doctor that specializes in heart, lungs and kidneys. This practitioner came to the facility weekly. pharmacy. If there is a particular pharmacy that is less expensive, talk with the D.O.N. about possible using your pharmacy of choice. But know that the family will be responsible for picking up medications and delivery to the facility. It is just in the best interest of the resident and family to use the facility's pharmacy. Just saying. That is my personal opinion.

14. Transportation: Talk with your tour guide about if the facility provides transportation to and from procedures. There are a number of procedures that can not be taken care of at the facility level. You should know in advance who is responsible for taking the resident to and from those procedures. An example of one of those procedures is a colonoscopy.

15. Last Survey: Long term facilities that bill medicaid and medicare for their services are required to participate in an annual survey by the state. This is a very intense time when the state sends in a survey team to audit the facility. The survey team goes through the entire facility with a fine tooth comb to ensure that the facility is adhering to regulations mandated by the law to operate appropriately. This is being told to you because it is mandated that the facility make available the results of the last survey. You may ask your tour guide where they keep the "survey

binder" and if you may glance through it. It is public knowledge. I am just going to say this, any facility with "**a current tag**" that is called an "I J" (stands for immediate jeopardy) probably is not the nursing home for your loved one at that time. Immediate jeopardy is exactly what it says. One or all residents are in immediate jeopardy for potential harm or have been harmed. Just be mindful that error is human. Things unfortunately happen. The bigger picture to look at is did the facility correct the problem, put an action plan in place and was able to get the I J tag lifted.

16. Ombudsman: while on your tour,ask your tour guide to show you the posting of the Ombudsman. Their name and number should be posted. The Ombudsman is a designated person by the state to be a resident advocate. Not all residents have family or friends to advocate for them. Write the Ombudsman's name and number down. Give them a call and get their insight on the facility. They are another great resource to collect information about the facility. Now you may not be able to reach them on the first try. Keep trying, leave your name and number and a brief message for why you are calling on their voicemail. They will call you back.

8

ADDED BONUS: RESIDENT'S RIGHTS

I want to share with you a list of Rights for a resident in a nursing home.

- A resident has the right to be treated with respect.
- A resident has the right to be free from abuse and neglect.
- A resident has the right to be free from discrimination.
- A resident has the right to have a representative notified.
- A resident has the right to spend time with visitors.
- A resident has the right to be restraint free.
- A resident has the right to make complaints.
- A resident has the right to obtain information on services and the cost.
- A resident has the right to make a complaint.
- A resident has the right to participate in activities.
- A resident has the right to coordinate or participate in resident groups
- A resident has the right to have privacy

- A resident has the right to property
- A resident has the right to their living arrangements.
- A resident has the right to manage their own money
- A resident has the right to exercise their rights as a United States citizen.
- A resident has the right to proper medical care.

These rights are strictly enforced by the government and by facilities across the United States. These rights are very vague. For example: A resident has the right to be restraint free. Well, what is considered a restraint? Restraints are not just physical. Restraints are also chemical. An example of a chemical restraint is the medication Haldol. This is an anti-psychotic medication. It is used to treat schizophrenia. Schizophrenia is a mental disorder. One of the side effects of Haldol is drowsiness. The drowsiness side effect can be considered a sedative. Sedatives are chemical restraints. I am telling you all of this because there is more to each and every right of the resident. Maybe my next book will shed some light on these rights. Once you pick a nursing home, your next step is to know their rights and yours.

9

CONCLUSION

There it is. This is just basic information to get you started in the right direction. I am just a nurse that is extremely passionate about the elderly. These decisions are not easy to make. They can be very stressful. Hard decisions like this can take its toll not just on the family but for the elderly also. It can drain everyone mentally. If time is permitting I advise you not to rush into a facility. If you have loved ones that are getting up in age, start looking now. Get familiar with your local nursing homes by becoming a volunteer. Get yourself familiar with how it all works. Get familiar with the do's and don't in long term care. Get your loved one involved with volunteering. These residents that are in a nursing home love meeting people, sharing their life story and just having someone to talk to or play a game with them. There are certain things you have to do in order to become a volunteer. It's not as simple as walking into a facility and say " I am here to volunteer". But the process doesn't take long. For example, the facility has to complete a background check on any and all volunteers. This is safety for the residents. Facilities need volunteers especially for weekends. You do not have to commit to every weekend. Maybe just one Saturday or Sunday a month.

If my book has helped you or inspired you in any way, I would be so grateful if you left an encouraging review for the book on Amazon. Thank you for your time and I hope this book was helpful.

10

RESOURCE

Centers for Medicare and Medicaid Services. (2023, September 6). *Your Guide to Choosing a Nursing Home or Other Long-Term Services & Supports*. Retrieved February 4, 2024, from https://www.medicare.gov/care-compare/en/assets/resources/nursing-home/02174-nursing-home-other-long-term-services.pdf?redirect=true